BE SKINNY

HOW TO LOSE 1 POUND DAILY

Makaila Renee

An Original Kaila's Playhouse Edition
KILLEEN, TEXAS

Books published by Kaila's Playhouse

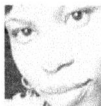

An original **Kaila's Playhouse** Edition
Baltimore, Maryland 21201

Copyright © 2018 by Makaila Renee

ISBN 13: 978-0-9974989-1-2

ISBN-10: 0-9974989-1-9

First Kaila's Playhouse printing- January 2013

Manufactured in the United States of America

Cover design by Makaila Renee

TABLE OF CONTENTS

Introduction
- A Commitment to Weight Loss .... **VII**

Common Weight Gain Factors ……..…………….... **9**
- Health Matters …………………...………… 13

Be Skinny Weight Loss Support System …..…...... **14**
- How to Use Be Skinny ……. ....…………... 15
- How Does Be Skinny Work? …………..…... 18
- Optimizing Be Skinny Results ………..…… 21

Be Skinny: Dietary Do's and Don'ts **23**

The Original Dr. Sebi Foods List …………..…... **25**

How to Prepare for Weight Loss …………….…... **29**

Additional Resources **33**

Be Skinny Quiz: Assess Yourself …………..……... **34**

Be Skinny Quiz Results ……………………..……… **37**

Works Cited …………………………...………… **39**

A BRIEF INTRODUCTION

This book serves as a manual and guide on how to lose 1 pound daily with Be Skinny Weight Loss Support System. The Ultimate goal of Be Skinny can be summed up in one sentence: A commitment to weight loss by natural means, for a natural body.

Unfortunately, toxins are everywhere we go. Toxins in the food, water, air and environment make cleansing our colon and organs difficult. This can have a debilitating affect on the immune system, which can affect weight loss. Although cleansing diets, herbs and fasting regimens have been around since the beginning of time, these natural remedies have been replaced with man-made, chemical filled alternatives, which can harm the body in the long run. While some popular diets come with prepacked meals, these processed foods are often packed with enough additives and preservatives to choke a horse. Not to mention the soy and other inflammatory agents waiting to be consumed by the unsuspecting dieter. Even weight loss pills and dietary supplements can contain toxic chemicals that can cause a chemical imbalance in the body. This means, no matter how strict the diet or vigorous the exercise, if you do not address the factors to weight gain, you will find it more difficult to lose weight- and keep it off!

What separates Be Skinny from other diets and weight loss programs is Be Skinny's ability to not only aid in detoxifying the body at the inner cellular level, but to identify and address key weight gain factors (like thyroid health, leaky gut, adrenal fatigue and low energy- to name a few), boost the metabolism, support digestion and decrease bloating and inflammation throughout the body, in order to heal the body and eliminate obstructions for optimal weight loss! After following the Be Skinny comprehensive manual on How to Lose 1 Pound Daily, you will feel better, look better and be up to 20 pounds lighter than before, GARUNTEED! Before you begin, you must first ask yourself:

Is Be Skinny for You?

To discover whether or not you are ready to embark upon the BE Skinny weight loss journey, feel free to take the Be Skinny self-assessment quiz on page 34.

Common Weight Gain Factors

Have you ever tried eating less and exercising more, but still haven't lost weight? Do you find yourself losing weight, then gaining it all back as quickly as you lost it? If this sounds familiar, Be Skinny Weight Loss Support System can help you solve these problems! To successfully lose weight, you must first pin point why you are gaining it. The most common reasons that most people gain weight can be attributed to what I call "weight loss factors". Weight loss factors include thyroid issues, adrenal fatigue, high cortisol levels, leaky gut, candida, cellular toxicity and lack of motivation. Be Skinny is a weight loss support system that helps to address each of these weight loss factors, so that you can finally burn stubborn fat and lose weight without wasting time, money and energy on strict diets, chemical-based supplements and/or strenuous exercising.

Thyroid Health 101

The *thyroid gland* (located right above the adam's apple) produces Thyroid Hormone (TH), which regulates body temperature, metabolism and the heartbeat, amongst other things. *Hypothyroidism* results from too little TH, or an underactive thyroid. Signs of an underactive thyroid can include low energy or feeling tired after a full night's sleep, depression, forgetfulness, low libido, dry skin, brittle nails (nails may have ridges), muscle pain, tingling or numbness in the feet, arms or hand (which may lead to nerve damage), thinning hair and weight gain. On the other hand, *hyperthyroidism* occurs when the thyroid gland produces too much TH, and is overactive. Signs of an overactive thyroid can include sleeplessness, feeling anxious or jittery, high blood pressure, thinning hair and weight gain.

Adrenal Fatigue 101

Adrenal glands are small (walnut sized) glands located above the kidneys that release hormones in response to stress. Too much stress or trauma can tire out or overwork adrenal glands. This is known as *adrenal fatigue*, although some people will simply say that they feel "burned out". Chronic stress can really take a toll on the body, leading to the breakdown of many systems within the body. Signs of adrenal fatigue can include mood swings, low sex drive or irregular periods, achy joints, tight shoulder or neck, premature aging, compromised immune system, trouble sleeping or staying asleep and weight gain.

In addition, *cortisol* (secreted by adrenal glands) can be too high which causes higher insulin levels and lower blood sugar levels, so you crave more sugary and fatty foods, resulting in weight gain. Adrenal fatigue can lead to the development of disorders like diabetes, heat disease, auto immune disorders (arthritis and hypothyroidism), gut disorders (leaky gut and irritable bowel syndrome), hormonal imbalance and obesity.

Leaky Gut 101

Leaky Gut Syndrome occurs when the "net" in your digestive tract get damaged, allowing proteins, gluten, bad bacteria and undigested food particles to leak from the gut lining and pass into the bloodstream. Leaky gut is caused by inflammation due to reactions to food and imbalanced bacteria in the digestive tract. Because insulins job is to burn calories to create energy, decreased insulin function means that your body will store fat as energy instead. In addition, increased cortisol levels will further decrease insulin levels and cause more leaky gut, thus perpetuating the problem, leading to the growth of candida (yeast) and causing bloating and weight gain.

Candida 101

Candida is a fungus that normally lives in the body (in small amounts) that aids with nutrient absorption and digestion, when in proper levels. An imbalance of bad bacteria in the gut caused by candida (yeast) can slow down the metabolism and disrupt the body's natural detoxification process, resulting in the release of toxins into the bloodstream. One of the many unwelcome signs of candida overgrowth is weight gain or difficulty losing weight.

Constant Fatigue 101

When your energy levels are constantly low regardless of how much you sleep, there is a strong possibility that you may be affected by one of the previously discussed weight gain factors. Dieting, hormones, candida, leaky gut, adrenal fatigue, cellular toxicity and thyroid disease can all affect low energy levels, motivation and may be the primary cause of constant fatigue.

Health Matters

No matter how much you diet or exercise, until you address the root causes to your weight gain, you will find it very hard to meet your weight loss goals on a permanent level. Friends, I tell you that we can eat all the fruits and vegetables that exist in the land, but if we do not heal of adrenal and thyroid gland and detoxify or blood, all of our effort may be in vain. The good news is that now that you have become aware of common weight loss factors, you can better understand why health matters are so important to successfully lose weight. In continuing to read this manual, you will soon discover how BE Skinny Weight Loss Support System can help!

Be Skinny Weight Loss Support System

Be Skinny is a completely natural weight loss support system that not only targets key weight loss factors, but also helps to heal the body by reducing bloating and inflammation, boosting and speeding up the metabolism and aiding proper digestion. Be Skinny contains some of the most powerful herbs from around the world to support weight loss and detoxify the liver, kidneys, gallbladder and purify the blood. What makes Be Skinny so effective is its ability to strengthen and heal the gut, thyroid and adrenal glands, lower cortisol, balance sugar levels in the body, eliminate candida and flush the colon, so you can lose weight- and keep it off!

Be Skinny Weight Loss Support System comes complete with everything that you need to start your journey to a healthier and fit lifestyle:

Be Skinny Weight Loss Factors (90ct)
Be Skinny Bloating & Inflammation (90ct)
Be Skinny Metabolism & Digestion (90ct)
Be Skinny Apple Cinnamon Tea (4oz)
Be Skinny Ginger & Cayenne Tea (4oz)
Be Skinny Hibiscus & Grapefruit Tea (4oz)
Be Skinny Licorice Tea (4oz)
Be Skinny Peppermint & Anise Tea (4oz)
Dr. Sebi inspired Detox Tea (5 gallons)
Colon Flush (30ct)

How to Use Be Skinny

Be Skinny Weight Loss Factors should be taken once daily. Take 3 capsules all at one time on an empty stomach or with food. Wash Be Skinny Weight Loss Factor capsules down with one full glass of spring water or Be Skinny Teas. Remember to drink at least ½ gallon – 1 full gallon of spring water of Be Skinny Tea daily.

Be Skinny Bloating & Inflammation should be taken once daily. Take 3 capsules all at one time on an empty stomach or with food. Wash Be Skinny Bloating & Inflammation capsules down with one full glass of spring water or Be Skinny Teas. Remember to drink at least ½ gallon – 1 full gallon of spring water of Be Skinny Tea daily.

Be Skinny Metabolism & Digestion should be taken once daily with the largest meal of the day. This means, if you usually have a big breakfast, and a light dinner, you will take Be Skinny Metabolism & Digestion with breakfast. If you enjoy a light breakfast and a big dinner, then you will take Be Skinny Metabolism & Digestion with dinner. Take 3 capsules all at one time with your meal. Wash Be Skinny Metabolism & Digestion capsules down with one full glass of spring water or Be Skinny Teas. Remember to drink at least ½ gallon – 1 full gallon of spring water of Be Skinny Tea daily.

Be Skinny Weight Loss Support Teas are composed of five unique blends of teas that you will drink with every meal. To prepare the tea, boil spring water, then add as much or as little of the powdered tea blends as you like. Turn off the stove and cover the pot with a top. Allow the tea to seep for at least 5 minutes (minimum). You can drink Be Skinny Teas hot (plain or add agave) or you can store the tea in an empty container to refrigerate and drink cold. If you chose to store Be Skinny Tea in the refrigerator, be sure to drink the tea within three days. Always make sure to have fresh limes handy for all your Be Skinny Tea formulas! DO NOT ADD SUGAR!

Dr. Sebi inspired Detox Tea and Colon Flush comes with directions on the labels. Follow the written instructions on the package to prepare the tea. You are to take three (3) Colon Flush capsules daily, all at once with the Dr. Sebi inspired Detox Tea. You may drink the Dr. Sebi inspired Detox Tea hot (plain or with agave) or you can refrigerate to drink cold. Drink Dr. Sebi inspired Detox Tea as often as you like, or as a three day power cleanse (prescribed below).

- 3 Day Power Cleanse with Dr. Sebi inspired Detox Tea:

Two (2) teabags make one full gallon of tea. Prepare tea as instructed on the package. Drink one half gallon of Dr. Sebi inspired Detox Tea with three (3)

Colon Flush capsules on the first day. Drink two cups of Dr. Sebi inspired Detox Tea with three Colon Flush capsules on day two. Drink two cups of Dr. Sebi inspired Detox Tea with three Colon Flush capsules on the third and final day. You can do the 3 day power cleanse every week.

How Does Be Skinny Work?

Be Skinny Weight Loss Support System works by targeting and eliminating key weight loss factors, so that you not only improve your health, but can successfully lose weight- and keep it off!

Be Skinny Weight Loss Factors (90ct) is packed with powerhouse herbs that address the gut, thyroid and adrenal gland health, promote healthy cortisol levels and curb candida overgrowth. Be Skinny Weight Loss Factors include, but are not limited to, rhodiola rosea and licorice root. Both herbs are adaptogens, or herbs that have a normalizing effect on the body to bring the body back to a balanced state. Adaptogens also help the body better adapt (hence the name adaptogen) to stress. Licorice root prevents the accumulation of fat by decreasing levels of SREBP-1 (a protein that promotes the production of fat) and increases levels of PPAR-alpha (which stimulates the breakdown of fats). Rhodiola Rosea, or rhodiola is also great for weight loss. According to a controlled placebo study done on 130 overweight patients in Georgia State Hospital, rhodiola extract led to a mean weight loss of 19 pounds, compared to only 8 pounds of loss by the placebo group who ate the same diet. Rhodiola also has tremendous fat burning, energy boosting power, can heal your thyroid, balances cortisol levels, stabilizes blood sugar, lowers cholesterol and boosts the immune system.

Be Skinny Bloating & Inflammation (90ct) is a unique herbal blend of anti-inflammatory herbs, designed to reduce bloating and inflammation throughout the body. Key ingredients include, but are not limited to, bladderwrack and turmeric. Bladderwrack contains iodine, which feeds the thyroid gland and is a great herb for reducing swelling, bloating and inflammation. Turmeric is also great for inflammation. A 2009 study performed at Tufts University discovered that curcumin (the active ingredient in turmeric) suppresses fat tissue growth, has anti-inflammatory properties and is a powerful antioxidant.

Be Skinny Metabolism & Digestion (90ct) is comprised of the best and most effective herbs that have been tested to boost metabolism efficiency and support optimal digestion. Unfortunately, the older we get, our metabolism starts to slow down, making digesting certain foods more difficult. Thankfully, Be Skinny Metabolism & Digestion use key ingredients like dandelion root and ginger root to aid digestion and speed up metabolic function. Both herbs are also well known for their ability to boost the immune system, cleanse the blood, regulate sugar levels in the body and lower blood pressure. Ginger is best used for increasing body temperature and boosting the metabolism as much as 20% after eating, allowing you to burn more calories. Dandelion root is an effective blood cleanser (especially for the liver) that aids your body's natural detoxification process by helping to breakdown fats during digestion. A mild appetite suppressant, dandelion root detoxifies cells, stimulates bowel movements, fights cancer development and regulates blood pressure.

Be Skinny Teas (5 - 4oz bottles) support weight loss in several different ways. Natural herbs like green tea, watercress, papaya enzymes, cayenne, grapefruit and peppermint oils (to name a few) are only some of the well-known herbs and oils that have effectively withstood the test of time and have aided in weight loss for centuries. Each well blended tea compliments and reinforces the entire Be Skinny Weight Loss Support System and further addressing problems of weight gain, to correct these issues and heal the body.

Dr. Sebi inspired Detox Tea and Colon Flush has been added to the Be Skinny Weight Loss System to complete the natural detoxification process. The Dr. Sebi inspired Detox Tea and Colon Flush helps to rid the body of bacteria, parasites and toxins, cleansing the body at the inner cellular level and detoxifying the liver, kidneys and gallbladder.

Optimizing Be Skinny Results

To optimize results of the Be Skinny Weight Loss Support System, fasting weekly is crucial. Fasting should be done for three consecutive days in a row (or longer if you wish), or a minimum of two consecutive days with NO FOOD. You will drink spring water and Be Skinny Teas in conjunction with Be Skinny's all-natural weight loss support herbal supplements only. There are tremendous health benefits of fasting, but one of the best benefits of fasting is to give the digestive system a well needed break! With so many toxins, processed and unhealthy foods entering the body, the digestive system is constantly breaking down and digesting foods- even while we are sleeping. Then of course, we wake up and put more food into our system, never allowing the digestive system a moments rest. When we fast, we allow the body time to heal and repair other areas of the body because it's no longer busy with the digestive process. Once food is digested, your brain sends out a signal to fight off infections and diseases, repair damage, and detoxify the body. Adding Be Skinny Weight Loss Support Teas and supplements will assist in speeding up this healing process.

Other Benefits of Fasting:

- Improves body composition and fitness
- Improves mood

- Boosts metabolism
- Improves cardiovascular health
- Lowers blood pressure
- Lowers blood sugar
- Decreases inflammation
- Supports healthier skin (slows the effect of aging)
- Enhances recovery from injury
- Increases resistance to stress
- Cleanses and Detoxifies the body
- Supports fat loss

NOTE: For those working more strenuous jobs that require you to exert more energy, it is best to fast on your days off.

Be Skinny Dietary Do's and Don'ts

Unlike many strict diets that require specific foods and strenuous exercises, The Be Skinny Weight Loss Support System only requires that you refrain from four things:

Four Major DON'T'S (The 4 S's):

No Sodas, no Sugar, no Starch and no Soy.

1. **Don't Drink Soda**. This includes store bought juices, wine, beer, liquor, energy drinks or coffee. You should drink spring water and Be Skinny Teas or blend real fruits and vegetables in a blender of juicer ONLY!

2. **Don't Eat Sugar**. This means no processed sugar or products that contain processed sugars. You can substitute sugar with organic agave or date sugar. Keep in mind, processed sugar can be hidden in so-called "healthy" foods, like granola bars, protein bars and smoothies.

3. **Don't Eat Starch**. This means no bread, pasta or rice, unless listed on the Dr. Sebi Foods List (*see page 25*). Starch turns into sugar and sugar slows down the metabolism. You can substitute traditional grains, bread and flour with spelt bread, coconut or spelt flour, spelt pasta and other approved alkaline grains. (*see additional resources on page 33*).

4. **Don't Eat Soy**. Soy can be hidden in many products. Be sure to check labels for ingredients to see if the product contains soy. Soy causes bloating and inflammation.

Be Skinny Dietary DO's:

1. **Drink one full gallon of spring water daily** (1/2 gallon minimum). The more water you drink, the better and faster the herbs can absorb into the body and enter your bloodstream.

2. **Two Day Fast**. You are required to fast at least two or three consecutive days per week. This means that you will only drink spring water and Be Skinny Teas in conjunction with Be Skinny's all-natural weight loss support herbal supplements. When we fast, our bodies finally have the chance to rest and repair itself (*See Benefits of Fasting on page 21 & 22*).

NOTE: If you eat meat, be sure to eat wild caught fish or free-range chicken and turkey that are hormone free ONLY! You may also consider replacing hydrogenated oils (which cause cellular toxicity and inflammation), like vegetable, canola, sunflower and safflower oils with healthier coconut or olive oils.

The Original Dr. Sebi Foods List

Vegetables

- Amaranth greens – same as Callaloo, a variety of Spinach
- Avocado
- Bell Peppers
- Chayote (Mexican Squash)
- Cucumber
- Dandelion greens
- Garbanzo beans
- Green banana
- Izote – cactus flower/ cactus leaf – grows naturally in California
- Kale
- Lettuce (all, except Iceberg)
- Mushrooms (all, except Shitake)
- Nopales – Mexican Cactus
- Okra
- Olives
- Onions
- Poke salad – greens
- Sea Vegetables (wakame/dulse/arame/hijiki/nori)
- Squash
- Tomato – cherry and plum only
- Tomatillo
- Turnip greens
- Zucchini
- Watercress
- Purslane (Verdolaga)

Fruits

Dr. Sebi says, "No canned or seedless fruits."
- Apples
- Bananas – the smallest one or the Burro/mid-size (original banana)
- Berries – all varieties- Elderberries in any form – no cranberries
- Cantaloupe
- Cherries
- Currants
- Dates
- Figs
- Grapes- seeded
- Limes (key limes preferred with seeds)
- Mango
- Melons- seeded
- Orange (Seville or sour preferred, difficult to find)
- Papayas
- Peaches
- Pear
- Plums
- Prickly Pear (Cactus Fruit)
- Prunes
- Raisins –seeded
- Soft Jelly Coconuts
- Soursops – (Latin or West Indian markets)
- Tamarind

Grains

- Amaranth
- Fonio

- Kamut
- Quinoa
- Rye
- Spelt
- Teff
- Wild Rice

Natural Herbal Teas

- Allspice
- Anise
- Burdock
- Chamomile
- Elderberry
- Fennel
- Ginger
- Raspberry
- Tila

Spices and Seasonings

Mild Flavors

- Basil
- Bay leaf
- Cloves
- Dill
- Oregano
- Parsley
- Savory
- Sweet Basil
- Tarragon
- Thyme

Pungent and Spicy Flavors

- Achiote
- Cayenne/ African Bird Pepper
- Coriander (Cilantro)
- Onion Powder
- Habanero
- Sage

Salty Flavors

- Pure Sea Salt
- Powdered Granulated Seaweed
  (Kelp/Dulce/Nori – has "sea taste")

Sweet Flavors

- 100% Pure Agave Syrup – (from cactus)
- Date Sugar

Nuts and Seeds – (includes Nut and Seed Butters)

- Hemp Seed
- Raw Sesame Seeds
- Raw Sesame Tahini Butter
- Walnuts
- Brazil Nuts

Oils

- Olive Oil (Do not cook)
- Coconut Oil (Do not cook)
- Grapeseed Oil
- Sesame Oil
- Hempseed Oil
- Avocado Oil

How to Prepare for Weight Loss

Although there are several different ways to prepare for weight loss, the key to success is to always bear in mind that everything you are doing is to achieve your weight loss goal. Meditating on the ultimate goal of fitting into smaller clothes or even becoming healthy enough to enjoy outdoor activities with your family can help motivate you to stick to your weight loss plan. Here are a few steps that will keep you motivated and better prepare you for your weight loss journey:

1. Remove Unhealthy Foods- Bad habits can be hard to break. By removing unhealthy foods and drinks and replacing them with healthier alternatives, you are keeping triggers out of sight and out of mind, until you are strong enough to say no- and mean it!
2. Set reasonable Goals- If you set hard to reach or unrealistic goals and fail to meet them, you may lose motivation and give up. Simply saying, "My goal is to lose weight" is a lot more vague and will keep you less motivated than saying, "My goal is to lose 3-5 pounds this week," or "My goal is to be able to walk up a flight of stairs without losing my breath." Focus on small attainable goals that will be easier to meet and lead you to a healthier lifestyle.

3. Write It Down- You can start a weight loss journal which can include a list of weekly goals, document daily food consumption and/or exercise log. Documenting your progress is the best way to keep motivated and easily make adjustments to meet your weight loss goals.

4. Prepare by making sure that you have plenty of spring water and fresh limes for your Be Skinny Teas. You can also fill up on spring water or fruits and vegetables in between meals.

5. Fill Up- The problem with most diets is that they leave you feeling hungry. Be sure that you are filling up on the right kinds of foods. Spelt flour can be used to make bread and tortillas replacing traditional four. You can use spelt pasta, mushrooms and homemade spaghetti sauce to make a mean spaghetti (I do this often) that will fill you up and satisfy your taste buds. Fruit is also very filling and can curb cravings for sweets because it has high concentrations of water and natural (not processed) sugar.

6. Schedule in Physical Activity- You do not have to go to the gym to workout (unless you want to). There are plenty of exercises that can be done from right on the sofa. You can do leg lifts using 5-10 pound ankle weights, while you watch

television or eat a meal. Heck, you can even turn the music on and dance for a few songs. Nobody is telling you to throw your back out- just get up and move!

7. Prepare for Setbacks- In the past, no one at work ever offered to buy me lunch until I was fasting. Only when I was fasting and trying to give my system a break, would people pop out of the woodwork like ninjas with plates of my favorite foods. Prepare for times such as these by thinking up an appropriate response in advance, like "I'm still full from breakfast." Be sure to walk away as cordial and as quickly as possible, so that you do not renege on your weight loss plans. Also, if you know that you will be having a lunch meeting with a boss, client or friend, try thinking ahead about what you are going to order.

Additional Resources

There are about a billion and one resources online regarding the purchase and preparation of alkaline based foods and recipes. I will not complicate things for you. Here is what I recommend:

Food

Jet.com
A great resource for spelt flour, pasta and other alkaline foods.

Alkaline Recipes

Ty's Conscious Kitchen
A great resource for alkaline recipes

Exercise

YouTube.com
Search: Couch Workouts

Be Skinny Quiz: Self-Assessment

Circle the number beside your response. Add points to
determine your results to assess your success for weight
loss readiness.

A. How committed are you about losing weight?

      1.   Not at all committed
      2.   Somewhat committed
      3.   Very committed

B. What is the main reason that you want to lose weight?

      1.   To make people notice me
      2.   To look good for an upcoming event
      3.   To improve my health

C. How much weight do you plan to lose weekly?

      1.   Any amount of weight is fine with me
      2.   1-2 pounds per week
      3.   3-5 pounds per week

D. How often do you enjoy sodas, sweets or processed
    foods?

      1.   Very often
      2.   Not often
      3.   Hardly ever

Be Skinny Quiz: Self-Assessment (cont.,)

E. How organized are you?

   1. Not that organized
   2. Somewhat organized
   3. Very organized

F. How will you measure your success for weight loss?

   1. My doctor will inform me of my weight loss progress.
   2. I will use a scale to weigh myself often.
   3. All of the above

G. How do you feel about exercise?

   1. I would prefer to lose weight without exercise.
   2. I don't love it, but I know I should do it.
   3. I exercise as much or as little as time allows.

H. How will you take dieting into your own hands?

   1. I will buy prepackaged meals and sugar free snacks.
   2. I will eat the same, but control food portions.
   3. I will prepare healthier meals and am willing to give up certain foods altogether.

I. How would you describe your current lifestyle?

   1. Very busy and stressful
   2. Busy, but not stressful
   3. I have at least an hour or two that I can dedicate to my health goals.

Be Skinny Quiz: Self-Assessment (cont.,)

J. How often do you drink soda, coffee or store-bought juices?

    1. Often
    2. Somewhat often
    3. I prefer water.

K. How often will you weigh yourself while using the Be Skinny Weight Loss Support System?

    1. Every 30 days
    2. Weekly
    3. Daily

L. If your spouse of co workers order a pizza, will you eat it while using Be Skinny Weight Loss Support system?

    1. If I like the toppings, I will definitely eat the pizza.
    2. Mabey, I will eat a slice or two.
    3. I will not eat the pizza.

M. After you reach your desired weight loss goal, what will you do?

    1. I will go back to my old diet, but if I start to gain weight, I will go back to eating healthy again.
    2. I will cut myself some slack, but still try to maintain my weight loss.
    3. I will continue to eat healthy and maintain physical activity whenever possible.

N. How do you feel about herbal medicine for weight loss?

    1. I think that prescription medication made in a lab, might work better for weight loss.
    2. I don't know much about herbs, but I am open enough to give them a try for weight loss.
    3. Herbal medicine is a natural way to help the body in a lot of ways, including weight loss.

Be Skinny Quiz Results

Results of final score:

35- 42 = Your motivation and level of commitment towards weight loss is excellent. You demonstrate that you are more than willing to do what it takes to lose weight and change your lifestyle on a more permanent level. Your odds of meeting your weight loss goals are very high, and you are sure to be successful, possibly even exceeding your weight loss goals.

21- 34 = Your motivation and level of commitment towards weight loss is solid. The idea of what it takes to lose weight may not thrill you, but you are definitely willing to do what it takes to live a healthier lifestyle. The odds of meeting your weight loss goals are good, and you are very likely to be successful.

14- 20 = You need to step your game up! Your motivation and level of commitment towards losing weight is very low. In order to successfully lose weight, you will first need to reassess your health priorities and carve out some time which should be dedicated to furthering your weight loss goals.

Less Than 14 = This may not be the right time for you to embark on your weight loss journey, but don't give up. You can always prove this quiz wrong and beat the odds!

Works Cited

Body Ecology, Is Your Weight Gain Tied to Adrenal Fatigue? 3 Steps to Recover Your Energy and Shed the Pounds

Dr. Axe, The Leaky Gut Diet and Treatment Plan

Doctor Doni, Unexplained Weight Gain- Can It Be Leaky Gut?

Global Healing Center, 20 Health Benefits of Fasting for Whole Body Wellness

WebMd, Can Stress Cause Weight Gain?

Works Cited